It's like I'm trying to find perfection, it's an ache that never goes away and it's a complete, total mind cluster. I mean it never stops. Every day it's like I don't know how my head is going to react, I don't know what's going to happen and I'm going to try to be someone different to accommodate . I'm so scared to be myself it's galling. Why am I trying to be someone for everyone? Why am I trying to be twenty different versions of myself? Why can't I just.. be myself? I mean surely that's how it should be right? I mean it's not a radical concept, it's not new, it's not ground-breaking it's just how I should be. This isn't hard, I'm making this hard.

I've been writing again, I bought myself a little book a couple of months back so I could document how I felt day to day, it started off well and within three days my mind went to shit. As always it started in a pub, shock horror of all shock horrors. It started off with me reviewing my previous workings, reviewing and thinking.. Then thinking and thinking, then thinking and over-thinking, couple all of that with alcohol and you have a perfect storm. I don't mean to be the person I am and I mean that, I know I have a lot going for me, it's why I have lots of people around me, lots of good people but the wiring inside my head seems to be getting more and more tangled but I'll come back to this later. I've decided writing this there will be no chapters, I don't want to be organised in my writing of this because quite frankly I want to speak from the heart here. I'm not saying the last two weren't written from the heart but after reading them and re-reading them I just don't feel they've captured what I want to say. Don't get me wrong I read them back and yea' they say a lot and I'm glad they're written but I'm missing something, there's something that's just not out, something that still eats away at me, something that slowly corrodes any happiness I build up and that is what I'm searching for. Whoever or whatever you are come out..

please come out..

So less than a week after finishing my second work I started writing again, I thought that if I kept my writing up I could better control all that goes on inside my head, in a way I think it did but the bad days I had at the start of June were really bad, I mean **REALLY, REALLY BAD.** Words like 'dysphoria', 'disaccociation', 'psychogenic amnesia' and 'de-personalisation' were present, I had shut down again and once again I was beginning to enter the abyss of depression and whenever that occurs it's inevitable that thoughts of suicide start to stir again. I feel I've gotten to a point with this that these types of thoughts are normal. I mean in my head they are normal because they're there that often it's just something I manage. In fairness I have been managing them well, I always find it easier to focus on my negatives as opposed to my positives though. I've always been the same, I've tried to change it but it's a hard habit to shift. I'll be upfront though and I will say I know it doesn't help me, focusing on negatives is never going to lead to a clean, healthy mind. Am I over-thinking again? Is this something that I should be seeking professional help over? Well, yea' the answer to question two is definitely a yes, question one I'm still contemplating over. I'll come right out with this right at the start so there are no misconceptions, I'm an alcoholic and it's something I will publically admit that I'm fighting,

I've been hitting the bottle **hard** and that is something I've found hard to beat, I've found it hard being sober outside of work, drinking is what I do, it's how I've 'coped'/'dealt/ with the inner workings of my head, yip I know, it's not the way to deal with it but I have no real other interests to speak of. I just don't get why my life is so hard, there's no reason for it to be as hard as this, I mean there just isn't, I have a great setup but it's my head, it's what goes on between the ears that's causing my life to be all convoluted and distorted, it's not having that simplicity, that peace of mind, that little bit of peace inside to just enjoy things, I mean it's something I'm craving, I'd quite like to sleep more than what I do, I'd like to worry less than what I do and most importantly I would definitely like to drink less than I do. It's only because I've ran out of money this month (July 2015) that I've stopped drinking, pathetic eh? The thing is though is I'm at my happiest when I'm on my own drinking, reading that I think it's going to look like a contradiction but it's really not. It's the one thing I like doing because it allows me to tap into what I believe is my right mind and start dissecting all that's happening, there is a fine line I'll admit but it allows me to write and write and write, it can't be right... can it?

It's hard though, I mean it's hard getting up in the morning when I'm having one of 'those days', the thing is they can come out of nowhere, it's like being side-slammed in a car and still having to go about my day as if everything's fine, that's the hardest part, that is **by far** the hardest part. I really don't want to have to fight this until I die but the thing is I think I'm going to have to. A thing that doesn't help me and it's entirely my own fault is I'm getting to the stage where I dreaded getting to. I've always said I didn't see myself getting past thirty-five I'm now thirty-three (and a half) and that age is looming, it's on the horizon and I hope that I not only see it but I live long after it. See stuff like that just isn't right but it's the way I think, I think at a very deep level and the way I see things confirms that to me. I don't look at things black and white, I see no grey areas I just see things as they are. Reading that back that sounds arrogant, it's not supposed to be it's simply meant to be a descriptive way of me trying to let you in. I need to let you in because if you see what I see then maybe you can see what I have to see, you see? To be honest I don't know if I'll ever be able to do this, I don't know even if anyone cares, I mean I'm just me, I am one insignificant person out of around seven billion, who cares really? I mean does anyone? I know I do and that's another part of my problem, I care WAY too much for everything. I don't have an off switch, I don't have the ability to zone out, I'm always on and I inevitably burn out from time to time, it's ok. I accept it. That's not to say it's all bad, I'm not trying to paint on a dark, depressive canvas, if that's the impression you get then I apologise, I'm not. I'm trying to paint a picture, an insightful picture. I'm not good that way, I don't really have the confidence to be myself, I live in my own bubble way too much, I hate it but when I come out of it, I just don't feel right.

If I keep searching will I find an answer? If I keep digging will I find a breakthrough. If I keep writing will I uncover a truth and if I keep questioning and I do find what I'm looking for will I like what I find? Ultimately what am I trying to achieve, am I writing just to vomit out all I suppress, am I trying to reach people? What am I trying to do? Can I be honest? I actually don't know, what I do know is that I'm trying to turn my mind inside out so I can have some peace, I deserve that much at least. I mean, there are times where I literally cannot function, there are times where I'm sat at the edge of my bed, looking out the window and I feel as if I'm actually trapped, I feel trapped both inside my head and inside my surroundings. I sit for hours and do nothing but stare, my head is too weighed down to do anything else. I put music on and I just sit. I don't reply to texts, I come off social media and I just.. sit, it's strange though because although I'm not allowed (by my mind) to do anything it's actually really calm inside my head, things make sense and I'm allowed to breathe, I sit and stare but nothing happens inside my head. It's actually quite nice because it gives me a rare break from vortexing thoughts, worries and over-thinking. The hardest thing about is being around people when it happens though, I can't speak to them, I have no choice in it, I just have to sit and focus on whatever task I'm doing, I'm limited to one-word answers and just endless focus and concentration, I find it hard to look in one place walking. I put music on and I find myself gazing skywards, looking at clouds, I find myself looking from side-to-side and then down, then back up again, I'm lost in the music, it's almost like the music is coursing through my veins, I walk in complete rhythm to the song I'm listening to, my thoughts align with the rhythm and my head movements align with the pace of my walking AND the rhythm. It's actually quite surreal, I could walk for hours, I could write for hours and I can be at peace for hours. I can disappear, I can lose myself inside myself for days and just not care about anything else, I go back to sitting on my bed and looking outside the window again, it is actually a sweet place for me to be but I know I can't stay there too long, if I do I'll just never come back from it. I need to come back from it.. (wake up Dave, time to return)

I'm terribly insecure in my appearance and my body, I never have liked how I've looked, it's just my way, I don't like myself that much, I'm pretty sure there's a link between that and my mental states, I just can't link them together. In fairness I am getting better at liking myself, it's something that's going to take a lot of work but I genuinely believe I work better being different from everyone else, I'm not good as 'another face in the crowd', I do like to be different and I'm in the middle of being that, it's a work in progress and as of today (12/07/2015) it's coming on fine, I just need to keep working on it, I'd like to point out I'm talking appearance wise, mentally I would love nothing better to be 'another face in the crowd' but at the moment I've got my appearance and my mental states the wrong way round. If I get the appearance bit right then I think the mental state will start moving in the right direction. That's the theory anyways, in practice I doubt it'll be that simple. I can dream though eh?

I'm actually really impressed with myself, two-thousand words and not one single swear word, considering just how much I swear that is a feat. I make Gordon Ramsay look polite when I get going, can I write this and not swear once? Tall order but I'll give it a go. One of the many problems I have is my sheer inability to understand/perceive people. I can never just be one of the gang and just have a laugh, even when I do my head manages to mess things up, I actually think it's better for me to be on my own because then it's me and my mind, we can work our differences out and then if we can't then the only person it affects is me. I can write, I can lie down, I can have a bath, I can go for a walk, I can deal with it on my own and there are no casualties, people then don't have to worry about me, I **HATE** people worrying about me and I'll explain why:

I appreciate the fact people care about me, I really do but I don't think it's fair on the people I love. I also don't like getting compliments, I really don't because I don't react well to them, once again I don't know why that's the case all I know is that it happens and I need to just deal with it. I find it tremendously hard to talk to people naturally, I always find myself struggling for words that sound right, I find myself grabbing sentences just so I can stay in a conversation and I don't like it, actually scrap that, I hate it. I strongly dislike the fact that I have to deal with this, I strongly dislike the fact that this takes over me and I just wish it would end. I don't wish my life would end but I wish this never ending tirade of mental abuse and violation would end, I honestly and genuinely think sometimes about running away, I think about where I could go to escape this but I know I never will. Maybe if I get my passport sorted, save up some money and then fly away I'll leave my mental capitulations behind, maybe if I start a new life then whatever mental problems I have to deal with will magically dissipate and I'll be happy, then I have to stop myself from thinking that way because I know that'll never happen and the longer I think of it the worse it's going to be when I'm dragged back to reality. See a lot of people dream for financial security, a lot of people yearn for 'the one', people dream of all sorts of things and you have to have a dream, if you don't have a dream then you're doing life wrong, everyone needs something to aspire to, something to achieve, to work for, strive for. My dream is to live in a mind that has minimal clutter, a mind that doesn't pollute the simplest thought, the simplest gesture, a mind that takes the good and shreds it into a million tiny pieces. I dream of living in a mind that is not only strong and robust but also allows for mistakes, a mind that allows things to happen naturally without setting off alarms, I YEARN for a mind that is free of breaking me down, wearing me down and shutting me down. I dream of having a mind that allows me to just simply be me and this is why I keep fighting, maybe one day I'll get my dream. I need to keep fighting, I WILL... keep fighting. Oh by the way on a side note the celibacy didn't last, I ended up having sex, oops. My intentions were good, just unfortunately my mind wasn't.

Do I need a change of scenery? Do I need to change myself? Actually do I need to change anything? I tried therapy before but I got scared and ran off. Maybe I need to try harder, I've already came so far so is it mind over matter? Mind over mind? Mind over MY mind? How can I make my two frames of mind one, I've had it before but can I have it again? I'm pretty sure it's achievable, it has to be, I mean it's not impossible, it can't be. There's no way I can spend the rest of my life focused on my mind, I mean if I do that then I won't be living, I'll be managing thoughts and that's not living. I... I don't want to exist, I want to live, I'm thirty-three, (and a half) there's got to be something for me, has anyone seen the switch? You know the switch, the off switch, it's around here somewhere, I need to find it so I can enjoy life. It can't be healthy living like this, actually scrap that, it's not healthy living like this. It breaks my heart, I mean it honestly, one hundred percent breaks my heart to have to constantly fight something that exists only in my mind. I've hit the bottom, I've tried to commit suicide and it failed, I've hit the bottom so now I should be swimming for the top, swimming for the top of the water, I should be looking upward but yet I continue to waste my gaze looking sideways. Is this my life? Is it the mental rollercoaster, am I always going to be eternally looking up then down, I really hope not. I really hope that I live my life, I mean the desire is there, the hunger is there and the burning is there. There is fire in my heart, blood pumping through my veins, light in my eyes and desire coursing through every artery within me, like all things with me though I know this is temporary, I know this will disappear and I know at some point the darkness will be back, it's always there, just out of sight and blocking the light at the end of the tunnel. I've grown to hate it, manage it and hate it. I need an identity, I need to formulate a plan that allows me to keep my head in check, at the moment I feel as if I've got it on a leash that's a rotting rope, I don't feel I have any control over my mind and that's just not healthy for me. The thing is though I've tried not thinking, I've tried free-wheeling and just not putting any thought into my head and it just doesn't work, if anything I feel worse for doing that. I mean is any of this making sense? I'm not sure it is, oh well best keep going.

It's like a weight, a weight that drags my eyesight down so I can't face myself in a mirror, a weight that causes me to constantly look down, to not be able to make eye contact with those I love. It's a weight that takes any happiness I have and anchors it so I can't reach it. In fact it's not 'like a weight', it is a weight, it pushes my head to my shoulders and makes day-to-day tasks an achievement should I achieve any. I remember I once went over forty days when I was at the height/depths of my depression, that's the hold this weight has over me. It makes even the most mundane, easiest tasks a chore, I have to reach deep down inside to have a bath, brush my teeth, cut my nails. I mean it has a hold on me, it has a vicious hold on me this and I wish it would just leave, I have no patience for it, I have no reason for it and I'm darn sure I have no desire for it. I'm at a point in my life where I feel like I'm a lot happier, I feel a lot more comfortable in my own skin and although I'm not one hundred percent I know it's getting there, I know I'm getting there and I see a lot more light than I used to. All in all I believe I'm coming out the other side, I keep pushing and fighting for it. It's a scrap but as someone that's used to fighting for things it's ok, I'm accustomed to it. I'm used to it and I'm going to give this everything I have, it just strikes out of nowhere though, the weight just clamps my legs like cement galoshes and just drags me under, leaving me at the bottom again and dreaming of swimming upwards again. It happens so quick, it cold-cocks me, it nullifies me, it takes anything good and turns it into a wretched, dehabilitating, numbing wreck of swirling thoughts. It somehow manages to find buried memories from my past, memories that I've fought so hard to deal with and it exhumes them. Infact it not only exhumes them but it resurrects them and places them right at the front of my mind again, when that happens I need to go into my cocoon, I need to ride it out and then I need to start the fight all over again.

Starting from the bottom of the ocean takes a lot of preparation. Once 'the weight' lifts from me I can then start my fight again, I see it go, I see it float away, I know I'll see it again, I know I'll have to fight it again but for now it's released me so I can chip away at the galoshes and then start swimming again, there is no pattern to this, believe me I've tried watching it, I've tried it, monitoring it, looking at weather, diet, alcohol consumption and there is no pattern. Sometimes it just strikes, sometimes it hits, hurts and punches. Sometimes it beats me, sometimes it violates me and it ALWAYS floors me. It's like the flu only you can't see it. I see it, I see it from the bottom. I see my friends and family above, I see them above the surface, I see them clearly, I reach for them and I know I'm miles away, I know I'm not going to reach them, I know I shouldn't try to but I need to. I'm trapped again, I'm under again, sometimes they're just out of reach and other times I just can't see them. Even when I sleep I suffer, I don't rest, I never rest and I get up the next again day, I get ready to face the day even though I'm not ready. It's at times like this I think about running/swimming away. Maybe the change of scenery.......

Yea' I know, it's never going to happen, I've accepted it and I've just got to accept it and await 'the weight'. It's funny, the worst part isn't when it hits the worst part is knowing it's going to, it's those two or three days of the thoughts mutating and taking on their evil forms, it's the feeling that the swirling has started and bit by bit the light is going to disappear, it's the preparations of the galoshes, the edging closer to the cliff, the look down at the water and the recognition of the spot where I'm going to be again. It's the realisation that soon enough I'm going to be searching for my friends again, I'm going to have to cocoon, I'm going to see nothing but black. It's the feeling of being trapped that disgusts me, I can take being quiet, as I eluded to earlier I actually quite like it, it's peaceful and actually provides me with some serenity, it doesn't always. Sometimes it double bluffs me and my serenity and peace are eaten away by the vortex, sometimes it leaves me nothing. It's a hurricane and destroys anything and everything positive in my path. The water I'm trapped in is so cold, my head is so heavy, people are talking but I can't hear anything, people are laughing and I can't hear anything, people are around me but I'm not seeing them. All I see are the two blocks at my feet holding me at the bottom of the ocean, I'm waiting on the weight again, I'm just waiting for it to come below the water and leave me there again, leaving me to fight again. I've lost count of the times I'm left alone at the bottom wondering if I'm ever going to win, I've lost count of the times I've craned my neck skywards crying at the thought of having to deal with this. I've lost count of the amount of times I have felt susceptible, vulnerable, the times I've felt exposed, open, bared and unprotected to this. I have well and truly lost count of the amount of times that this has violated me and caused me to take on a whole different form, the amount of times I've lashed out at friends, I know it's not me but it disguises itself as me, guys it's not me, I'm trapped, lost in ocean of my own thoughts, please you need to understand this person that's snapping and faltering is not me, IT'S NOT ME. Guys help, can you hear me? I'm trapped, I'm lost, I'm drowning here, look it's me. I'm here you can't hear me though can you? I'm trapped watching this, I'm a spectator to my own destruction, I'm powerless and helpless. On top of everything else I've now got to watch myself implode, I hate it so much, it takes up so much of my time and takes up all of my resources, I am stretched to breaking point and does he care? Does it care? Of course it doesn't because it's doing the one thing it's always taken great pleasure in doing. It's destroying my happiness, it's destroying everything I've built up from the last time it hit. It enjoys ruining me and it loves the fact I'm watching whilst it....

no... **_HE_** loves it, he laughs whilst I'm stuck there, sitting on the ocean floor, he sits above me and pushes me down, he makes sure I'm grounded, glued, fastened, stuck, welded to the floor. I sit with my arms crossed staring at the ripples that flow around me, the water is getting cold again, he 's been here too long, he's been here way too long, why does he want me to suffer? What does he get out of it? Why is my happiness his enemy? What have I done to him, what did I do? Did I hurt you? Did I embarrass you? Please tell me, talk to me and tell me what I've done, you're absolutely and completely destroying any iota of happiness I have, that's all I want so why do you take it away. I hate you, I hate you so much but why do I even tell him because all that does is give him more enjoyment over me. He leaves me shipwrecked, he leaves me a broken mess and when he does finally leave me to break out I've then got to start all over again. I don't see him for days, weeks, months, sometimes even years but the longer he leaves me the more devastating it is when he appears again. Sometimes I stave him off, sometimes I pre-empt him, I feel the presence, I feel the heaviness of my feet, I feel a shiver, I feel something, I feel him, he's there, he's watching, he's always watching me and I know I've got to be ready for him to strike, he's dragged me under so many times that I know when he's about now. I've got to be most aware when I'm at my happiest, that's when he picks his time to strike. I know it is, he knows me intimately, he feeds of my misery so why strike when I've nothing to lose. He knows the time to strike is when I'm at my best, he ignores the cyclic, he ignores my bad days because I'm suffering, he loves watching me suffer, writing anything and everything to try and escape, he loves the thought of me wanting alcohol, he loves the thought of me thinking of suicide, he absolutely loves it and he loves watching me fight. What truly makes him happy though is him taking everything away from me. He loves when I'm at my happiest and then that's when he strikes, he contorts, distorts and punctures me, he stabs me right in the head and leaves me to bleed out, he leaves me with nothing, HE... LEAVES...ME....WITH....NOTHING, **HE LEAVES ME WITH NOTHING,**

HE LEAVES ME WITH ABSOLUTELY NOTHING.

How many times have I been left to die at his hands? Too many to mention. The fact that nobody really knows this I think shows good management on my part, either that or I'm a really good liar, actually I know that's not the case I'm a terrible liar. He is there though. I know he is and I know he watches me. He's like ... what is he like.. He watches everything I do and he bides his time, he is the hunter and I am the prey. I've fought this long enough so when he strikes I know what to do when I'm at the bottom again. I'm going to leave him for now, just thinking about him makes me shiver, he's creepy.

So earlier I touched on writing just after I finished my second work, looking back at it it's scary how quick my thoughts changed, in the space of three days I'd went from writing things like 'Felt Good', this was on 30/05/2015 and within three days I was mapping these:

- Dysphoria
- Emotional Detachment
- Psychogenic Amesia
- Depersonalisation
- Introversion
- Splitting

This was three days worth of writing where I didn't speak to anyone, I had to be locked away within myself trying to get to the bottom of what was happening to me. This is why I always need to be aware, I mean things took a turn over what turned out to be about four days, I look back at the writings and I can actually see when things started changing, it's a little un-nerving but at the same time I know that I'm likely to see that whilst writing . I know when I write that more often than not something isn't right, I'm not going to be as arrogant to say it's like a sixth-sense it's just a feeling I get. Bear in mind between the ages of eighteen to twenty-nine I had filled about ten notebooks with writing, I mean that's all I done and I could count on one hand how many writings were happy. They weren't and a lot of them were very very scary. At one point I'd written a suicide note and this was in 2006. So even when I was twenty-four the demons were there, infact looking back I'm glad I did write, after 2011 when I nearly committed suicide I decided to get rid of them, I don't know if I done the right thing, I think I did but I don't know. Might have been nice to check in with them and see if what I was feeling was similar to what I feel now. I wonder if 'he' has always been there, was it him that started messing me up at eighteen, was it him that started me wanting to be alone? Hmmm, I wonder, the older I'm getting though the more he is interfering , the more he is taking control, the longer this goes the harder I need to fight to keep him out, I need to keep him out because one day he's going to get control of me and cause me and my loved ones a tremendous amount of pain. I'm fighting hard, I'm fighting super hard to manage my mind, I'm fighting to control my alcoholism, actually writing this I'm also fighting the urge to swear, still haven't though, this could actually be the longest I've gone without swearing.

There's something strange about trying to delve into your psyche, it's weird trying to tip it out for everyone to see, it's slightly off-putting but then I know in order for me to try and defeat/stave off this I know I'm going to have to. I know that it means I'm going to have to dig and already I know something I'm going to say that isn't going to be easy to read for me...

I need to be on my own, I need to stay off of social media and I need to socialise with people when I know that *HE* isn't around, he caught me out a few months back and I won't allow him to do it again, I can't allow him to catch me out. I need to do things on my own terms but whether I do that or not is anyone's guess, I think it'll be highly unlikely because I know myself that I don't follow-up on things, I don't learn, I'm not half the person I think I am because I keep falling into the same traps, I'll go out when I'm not feeling well, I'll have too much to drink and I'll end up blowing up. I'm not learning and that's stupidity, it's first-class idiocy and it irritates me. I'm not stupid, I'm way better than this and ultimately I need to start heeding the signs, it's ok me writing and saying this but I need to start doing it, I need to start taking my own advice, it's ok when I'm giving advice but when it comes to me actually taking any I don't. That's bad, I can't afford to do that with all that goes on inside my head, if I'm ever going to beat this then I need to start heeding both advice and the danger signs. So today (12/07/2015) I've taken myself off of social media, pretty sure I've done this before and failed but as I'm writing this I'm actually saying this to myself I NEED TO FOLLOW-THROUGH WITH THIS', me and social media do not get on, I NEED to take myself away from it and I need to focus on myself, the world doesn't need to know everything I do and I certainly don't need to know everything it does. I'd be quite happy not knowing what people are doing so if I take myself away from that it should help. The thing for me is can I stay off of it? I'll need to, it drives me nuts and I probably drive it nuts.

I need an identity, I need something to hold on to, I need to start work on being myself because at the moment I'm not. At the moment I alter my persona to fit in with people when I know I shouldn't, when I'm myself and this is in a working sense I'm very much tuned to my job, I find it easy to just get in and get stuff done, it's how I do things but I've found myself just inputting into conversations just for the sake of doing so. It's not right and I don't like it, I am so scared to be myself it actually sickens me a bit. There is nothing wrong with me being myself, I just get so scared to be it though incase people start thinking something's wrong and that's what messes me up. That sentence right there is a nail right on the head. I'm scared to be quiet (I'm naturally quiet) incase people think that something is wrong, that whole ethos is wrong, it's a crap theorem, it's a stupid equation, it's a totally crap way of looking at things, I'm better than that, that's why I need to start finding this clarity and peace of mind. If I don't I'm just going to think myself to an early grave and one thing I know for definite is this... **He** has absolutely nothing to do with this, this whole charade has been my own creation.

I think it started when I left school and I started work, in high school I done ok, I was neither popular nor bullied, I just got on with things. When I started work I wanted people to like me so I sort of faked my personality, so I'd go on nights out and pretend I was this total rock and roller who liked nothing better than boozing and shagging, don't get me wrong, I do like these but they're not all I am. I wanted to be popular, I wanted people to think when they looked at me, 'legend'. In hindsight I'd play it entirely different because after fifteen years of not being me it's began to fester away at me, it's began to eat away at me and now I'm going to find it hard to change. Then again a question I actually need to ask myself is this...

Who am I?

As in, who am I because I don't actually know. Don't get me wrong it's not through lack of trying or through lack of effort but I genuinely don't know the guy that's staring me back in the mirror. There are many reasons for that though, to an extent I've lost my way a bit, my judgement is clouded, I overthink things to death and I've allowed alcohol to control me, gone are the days where I enjoy the odd drink, I now drink whenever I can, that's sad and it makes me sad actually admitting that I'm an alcoholic, there are no two ways about it, I am and it's something I need to address, it's something that I have started addressing though but it's something I need to stay on top of. I need to stay on top of it because when I come 'off the wagon' I come off of it hard. I get bored easy, I'm currently back staying at the folks and I drink out of sheer boredom, god knows what's going to happen when I get my own place, I really need to build up my mental strength for when that happens, I know what I'm like and I know by a long way that alcohol is my biggest vice. It's not my only one though, the fact that I don't really know who I am is up there, I have no identity, I have nothing else to differentiate me from anyone, it's almost like I'm a zombie, I just seem to exist with no real purpose, one day merges into another, it's then a week, then a month and before I know it I'm another year older and it's yet another year where I've not done anything of note. It kills me, it really does, I mean I genuinely feel as if I'm wasting my life.. I mean am I? Am I wasting my life? It feels as if I am but then I think of all that I have to contend with, I've said it myself I don't feel as if I'm connected the way others are so am I wasting my life or am I fighting for my life? I should really know the answer to this but I don't, I don't have the answer, I don't have it. I mean…. why don't I have the answer? I don't even know what I want, do I want a girlfriend? Do I want lots of money? Do I want a nice house? I don't know, again I.. DON'T… KNOW. It almost feels like there's a part of my mind that's locked, like it's been hidden away. The core is there but when it comes to me trying to work out what I actually want I can't tell you. It saddens me, it really saddens me that I can't tell you what I want out of life, at the moment, short-term I'll take managing my thoughts and him. It's not exactly out of this world stuff though is it? I feel like I'm split into three different versions of me, the strong version, the weakened version and the reflective version. It's probably stating the obvious but the three parts never combine, each one makes up one third of me and at any one time only one part is in operation. Nine times out of ten it's either version one or version three that are in operation but when version two strikes it then the trouble starts. Although it's only one part of me the weakened version has various forms and versions and they range from under the weather to full on manic/depressive/suicidal forms, unfortunately when that version of me is operating it's hard for me to manage, I have to really grit my teeth and fasten my seatbelt because depending on the form I take even being around people takes a lot. It's a crippling state of mind to be in and I mean that. It manifests itself as different forms of depression and slowly but surely eats away at my strength. The only time I'm at the higher end of that scale is when '_he_' appears, when he appears I know that I'm in trouble. This has been the first time I've been able to humanise him, probably because he's been on my mind a lot since I went off from work last year with depression. Mind you it was coming for a long time last year, I'd basically hid it for months and my drinking sky-rocketed, when that kind of stuff happens things just aren't right. I'd managed to blow a substantial amount of money over three months and to this day I can't really tell you what I actually spent it on, that didn't help but you know what really didn't help? Not talking to anyone, hiding it, burying it so everyone thought I was fine, I wasn't fine, I was the furthest thing from fine. I was in so much pain that I was suppressing the manic/depressive/suicidal forms of myself, to be honest I don't know how I lasted so long, it must have been about three months of carrying on the charade that I was ok, yea', that worked out well didn't it?

I honestly wish you could see inside when I'm hit, see inside when I'm hurt. Physically there is no difference but mentally he caused me so much pain. Looking back I didn't realise just how much strength it took me to get through each day. Actually looking back I don't know how I managed to get through each day, there were a lot of days where I done nothing. I mean I done absolutely nothing. I spent my days either playing xBox all day and not moving or I spent the day wandering from room to room, I was almost in a catatonic state of mind, nothing was happening, I spent day after day sitting, I spent day after day looking out of my window, I spent day after day after day after day trying to figure out what this was. I spent so much time trapped in my mind that it changed the person that I was, I was trapped so much in my mind that I was not only at the bottom of the ocean when he hit me, by the end of December when I had my two suicidal episodes I was actually giving in to him. I had had enough of it. I spent over one hundred days chained inside my mind, I'd spent that long inside that I couldn't get out. By the time I had reached the middle of December I had no fight left, I'd fought and fought and I had nothing to give, it was by far the hardest thing I've ever done, by far the hardest decision I'd ever made but I'm glad I made it, it was the indicator I had reached the bottom and make no mistake. This wasn't a cry for attention, this wasn't me saying I needed help I want to make one thing painstakingly clear, that night I overdosed I fully intended on taking my own life. I had given in and I was tapping out, I had had enough, my mental strength by the end was paper thin, now for someone who prides themselves on their mental strength that is a hard thing for me to admit, I have no shame in admitting it though because after a lengthy battle I have to say I lost. By that time in mid-December I wasn't the same person, I wasn't the man that my family and friends knew, when I looked in the mirror I felt nothing, I had no care for myself, for weeks I knew I was running low on fight and the water was just below my chin, I felt the weight pulling and pulling and pulling and after fifteen years of wars I had eventually lost. The weights finally dragged me under and I began to slowly sank and drink my way to the bottom. I was drinking so much that I had lost the taste of beer, it was just a way for me to get away from my troubles, I was drinking so much in fact that it was routine for me to go to the shop and just buy six 660ml bottles of beer and just get drunk. I spent my final few weeks giving in and drinking my way to death, I'll admit it, I have to. I tried going online and pouring my heart out via online channels and making videos but it didn't help. By the end I wasn't even a shell of my former self, just a depressive alcoholic with nothing to take but pills. I took twenty-one pills all at once, I'd done it, I'd finally plucked up the courage to commit suicide, did it feel euphoric? No it didn't because after I'd done it I'd realised I'd given in, I'd succumbed, he had won and I could hear him laughing at me. I knew that by overdosing I had finally admitted he was stronger. I ended up in hospital vomiting as my brother had phoned an ambulance, twice in one week I'd ended up in hospital as only seven days previously I was one step away from jumping off of the balcony on my flat. Unless you suffer you can't possibly understand the sequence of events that take you there, that lead you there, the events and trauma and pain that slowly cut off every escape path and direct you to that. Unless you suffer then you'll never understand the thought of your very soul giving up and accepting that death is the only thing left. You'll never understand and if I can be one hundred per cent honest with you...

.. I wish I couldn't understand it either. Depression is one of the most horrible things that you can ever encounter, it's one of the most debilitating, destructive diseases that you can ever suffer from. Depression is an evil, demonic disease that causes you to take different forms. It's an absolute horror, what really gets me about it is I know that I've been doing better, yes I've had not so good days and a few bad days but I know I'm never going to beat it. I now know the rest of my life I am going to have to always be alert, I'm always going to be watching for the danger signs. I know that through my thirties, forties, fifties and sixties I am going to have to be vigilant. I wish I was an airhead, I wish I had nothing between the ears, I wish that my spelling was bad, I wish that I had nothing going on so I could live a life of ignorance. I absolutely hate the fact that I have to manage three differing versions of me and I really hate the fact that I can't talk to anyone about it. I've tried, god knows I've tried to but I just can't open up. I've said it before and I'll continue to say it but I cannot talk to people about this because I feel as if it's not real, I don't believe people will be taking me seriously when I say what I've said above. I want to be completely open about this and the only way I can do that is to write, I think this is the way I'm going to have to deal with it, by writing. In many ways I don't think that's a bad thing, infact in many ways I think it's actually a good thing because when I'm writing I talk no-holds barred, I talk with no filter, no fear and I talk openly, honestly and freely. The hardest thing for me is always going to be managing it when I have to be around people, it's awful when I'm on my own in a social environment and I just cannot talk, it's gut wrenching knowing I'm going to have to sit for two to three days knowing I'm going to be on my own. I get home and it's not any better there, when this strikes I never want to be anywhere. When I'm at home I want to be at work, when I'm at work I want to be playing snooker, when I'm playing snooker I want to be at home and so on and so on. It is absolutely horrible, my appetite goes right down, my alcohol consumption goes right up, I don't take care of myself and I make the biggest mistake of all.. I block people out. How do I talk to people when I don't know what to say? How do I call someone or text someone and say 'I need to talk' when I'm scared to death of what's going to come out. When it comes round I think of suicide, it's part of my thought pattern when this comes around, I can't help it and it annoys me. When I broke down at work last year I tried calling The Samaritans but I just couldn't. I tried but when you're bawling your eyes out it's really not fair on the other end of the phone, they're just not going to be able to understand. I tried though, I mean I genuinely did try. ☹

A lot of the paragraphs I want to start with 'do you know what my problem is' because a lot of what messes with my head is to do with me, there is very little outside that interferes with me and I'll give you an example. Today is Sunday, Sunday the twelfth of July, I finished work on Friday the tenth of July and I was looking so forward to the weekend, now that I'm on the weekend I'm looking forward to going back to work and I am ninety nine. nine percent sure that as this week goes on I'll be looking forward to the weekend again, my point being this. I absolutely suck at staying in the present, I'm either wishing my time away whatever I'm doing or when he strikes I'm constantly regretting every single thing I've done in my past, I hate it, I absolutely frickin' hate it, it's something I've worked on but I just can't seem to do it. I'm also way too harsh on myself when it comes to making mistakes, I allow myself to get away with absolutely nothing, I make a mistake and I replay it and replay it and replay it, it's ridiculous. I over analyse myself on everything I do, I don't like the way I look and I never really feel right in my own skin. I know I can't change that one and as I said earlier I am working on that but it will take time. My point being this, I shouldn't be looking back and if I do I should be proud but I'm not, I have this empty/nothingness type feeling going on and it's almost like I've been numbed by anaesthetic, it's a feeling that just has nothing attached to it. It's dull, it's boring and I'm sitting here looking at this thinking how much further do I need to hate myself before I start appreciating me for who I am. There's a lot I can't change about myself, my hair isn't going to grow back so I need to keep shaving my head, I can't change my age because as we all know time is a constant and stops for no-one, I can't change what's happened in my past so there is absolutely no point in dwelling and revisiting/regretting. The thing that I need to look at changing is my mindset, or do I? Ninety percent of the time I have the right mindset, I'm positive, hard-working, friendly, organised and in control, it's just that ten percent when I lose control that I need to change. In fact even that's not true because in general even when I have bad days I still manage to control them pretty well. I'm confused, I'm genuinely and utterly bamboozled as I sit and write this. I don't even know if my mind is tangled or untangled, I can't tell you how I'm feeling because like I say I'm almost numbed. I've done nothing today, I've spent all day in my pj's playing xBox and I feel relaxed but something inside me is telling me I should have done more, should I have done more though? I mean, it's a Sunday so I should have went on a bike ride or went for a walk, instead I've drank my weight in coffee and basically tried to once again make sense of this chaos that rages within me. I wonder sometimes if I'm ever going to be able to make sense of it. I wonder actually if I want to make sense of it. There has to be something to it, I mean... there's got to be.... right?

There's something that I always seem to come back to, a thought that always seems to be there no matter the train of thought. It's ever present with me and as today (12/07/2015) has gone on and the longer I've been off social media it's been growing..

'I'm better off on my own' and do you know something, maybe I'm right, generally I do work better on my own because any thought process that I go through tend to get worked out better on my own. I don't want this to be taken as I don't want to be around people but I think for the next wee while I'll stick to my own company, I think it's better that way and to be honest it's something I'm going to think about long-term, I need to be on my own for a bit, I think I get too involved with people and that's not where I need to be, plus taking myself off of social media is a good thing, I don't get on with it so you could say I've been proactive, you could but you probably won't. It doesn't matter, honestly. Am I depressive or is it that I just think at a deeper level than your average person, are the problems in my head medically related or are they caused by just how much I think? Obviously if I knew the answer to that I wouldn't be sitting writing trying to get to the bottom of it, I'd be sitting playing the xBox and not giving a toss about all of this, I only write when something is wrong and the fact that I've written nearly ten thousand words in less than five hours is giving me cause to think something isn't right or to put it more directly, it's making me think something is wrong. I said it earlier, looking back at my historic writing ninety five percent of it was when something wasn't right, all the little graphs I made and poems I wrote were all suggesting of something dark swirling through my head. All the previous writings pointed to feelings of despair, being unable to relate and a full-on assault against myself. Maybe I could run away, I mean... no-one would ever expect it. No-one would see it coming, obviously they would when you're reading this because basically it exposes the full detail of the plan but as I'm typing it it's definitely feasible. I need the silence of my own mind, I need quiet, I need lots and lots of quiet, there's too much goes on at my folks house in order for me to gather my thoughts, that sounds ungrateful but the longer this fight goes on the more I need to work out what I need in order to manage this, I've accepted I'll never beat this, that's fine, if I'm going to manage it though I'm going to need to surround myself with everything I need to get through this when it/he strikes. One thing I definitely need is my own space, I don't have that right now and I don't want this being taken as an excuse but I have been going out drinking, mainly because I need time to myself, it's one thing I desperately need right now and I just don't have it. God that sounds awful, I love my parents, I do and they are amazing. I just wish that I didn't have to deal with this. It's even harder to deal with when they're around, there are days I need to sit in silence, I don't have that option right now though.

The more I'm writing the more I think I'm learning to understand what goes on in my mind, I've read my first two back and although they're insightful I don't think they hit what I need to hit. Don't get me wrong, I'm not knocking what I've written but when I read them back I just don't feel like I thought they'd make me feel when I read them. I'm proud, I'm proud of the journey that I'm going through and I've accepted that my goal in life is knowing I need to find effective ways to manage it. I think I've done ok, yea' there have been times where I've not managed it well but I'm not a machine, I'm human, as much as there's a lot that goes on inside my head I do a pretty good job of managing this, this isn't easy, this isn't something that I particularly like having to juggle but I do and the fact that I manage it is something I take great pride in. Just sometimes it gets really hard to deal with, those are the days that I would gladly trade. I'd quite happily take the flu for four days rather than go through what I have to go through, the depths I have to plumb, the amount of sludge and slurry I've got to trawl my mind through, the sheer mountain I have to climb just so I can get through the day and then get to my bed. Even then when I get to my bed what happens? I lay awake and I think, I get about four hours sleep and then it's time to face it all again. I can't even tell you just how hard it is to get up on days like that, my legs weigh ten tonnes, my head weighs ten tonnes and my mind weighs about twenty tonnes, ugh, it's on those days I wish I was simplistic, on those days I feel as if I would be best served locking myself in my bedroom and just not communicating with anyone, that's not being dramatic, that's actually what I feel like on those days, the word brutal doesn't even do it justice. I keep thinking about getting professional help, I mean it's never really something that's far away from the front of my mind but I don't know the best way to go about it, besides the fact I don't feel comfortable talking to my closest about the war that rages inside my head so how the heck am I going to talk to a complete stranger about it. I mean maybe I just need to take the plunge and do it, I've got material behind me now that helps but I don't know, I want to... I'm just so scared.

(On a side note, ten thousand words and not one swear word, that's got to be the longest I've went without swearing)

I AM AN ALCOHOLIC

And I am, just writing it helps because I am. I don't drink to socialise, I drink to forget, I drink to escape and I drink just for the sake of drinking. It's a nasty thing to admit but I have to admit it, this is all about the truth and if I sit here and lie about it then I'm not going to get anywhere am I? I do use it as a coping mechanism and I do actually sometimes crave a pint. With a little resolve over the next couple of weeks I'm looking to reduce my alcohol intake as I need to focus on myself without booze, it does genuinely help me if done in moderation and I know it's a depressant, that's why I know if I drink in moderation then it does genuinely help me unwind, unfortunately though it's not always done in said manner and occasionally I do hit the bottle hard, I can't say I enjoy it much but I actually do it out of boredom a lot. As I stated earlier I get bored easily and it's just what I do, yes ok it's not ideal but it's something I need to manage, with me it's not really about enjoying life a lot of my time is spent managing the varying different things that go on in my life. God I feel as if I'm reflecting on my life thirty years too early, I'm reflecting and talking about regrets, jeezo I'm thirty-three, why the hell am I doing this? I'll tell you why I'm doing this is because I have to, I've said it before and I'll continually say it, I am not the same as your average person, my head does not operate as it 'should', it's something I'll say until I'm blue in the face, I won't apologise for it and I certainly won't shy away from it, I've spent way too long doing that, now's the time where I've got to face it head on. This is why I'm writing, this is why I'm delving, digging, unearthing, rearing, you name what I'm doing and I'm doing it. I want to get this all out so I don't need to write anymore, it's not even the fact that it hurts it's the fact that I'm missing out on so much because of my mind's inability to cope with the majority that it sees and feels, yet another thing I've always said is I feel my mind operates at a highly sensitised level, I feel a lot more, I feel compassion more, I feel empathy more and when all of that combines it unbalances me, it does it causes an imbalance in my head and that's what leads to the not so good days/the bad days and dare I say it, they lead to 'him'. I don't know if maybe I'm trying to fix something that's not broken or if I'm trying to fix something that's totally broken, this links back to what I was saying earlier, I just do not know what or how I feel, it's this big empty hole that just doesn't seem to be filled. I feel it, I feel things but it's almost like what's in my head over-rides the feeling if that makes sense? I feel, I genuinely feel but it gets numbed, it gets lost in the weight of my mind and then I don't know what I feel. It's hard, it shouldn't be this hard but it is. It's something I accept but it doesn't stop me from fighting it, it doesn't stop me wanting to be like everyone else and it will never stop me from trying to be like everyone else. Out of this I'm determined to live as normal a life as possible, I want to live my life and then die, I do not want to die and throw my life away...

.....if only it was that simple.

See, the fight and the hunger are there, the desire is there so I know I'm doing something right. I know deep inside this vault of a mind I've got it, I know it's there but I just need to unlock it, I need to fight through the weeds, the dirt and the mire to get to it. The good stuff's there, I've felt it before and I know it's there for me. I just need to find a way of getting to it and then keeping the bad stuff away from it. I don't use this line often but I deserve at least that much, I do, I've worked hard enough for it. I don't want to see hell or him again, quite honestly I've seen enough of both to last a lifetime, I don't need them anymore, I've seen the depths and the demons too much, I'm tired of seeing them, I'm focused on finding the good stuff again, the simple stuff, the nice stuff. The end of the working day and chilling with friends stuff. That's what I'm working towards, that's what I want from life, that's what I'm aspiring to, I want the simple things, I want the nice things. All I want are my friends, my family and the good times and as long as I'm breathing I'm going to fight for them. I need to fight for them because if I don't I'm not fighting for anything, I'm a man without a dream, a rudderless ship, a directionless wanderer destined to wander the rest of my life wondering, a 'what if' kind of guy, an 'If I'd only done this kind of guy', nobody wants to be that guy surely, I certainly don't. I want to do things, I want to travel the world, grow a big beard, get tattooed, spend quality time with friends and family, meet new people, become interesting. I want to do stuff, I want to see stuff, I mean that's not a lot to ask is it? I don't think it is to be fair. I mean it's achievable, I don't think what I've said there is the most ambitious set of life goals that anyone has set, I mean I'm never going to score the winning goal in a final or win the Nobel Peace Prize, I'm not being unrealistic here am I? In fact I think I'm being quite the opposite, I think I'm actually being quite realistic about the whole thing. It just comes down to being able to control my mind, that for me is the biggest challenge I face. Granted it's a pretty big challenge but definitely one I can win. What I'm trying to illustrate here is yes I'm not the biggest fan of my mind and yes I've got a lot to deal with but it doesn't stop me fighting and it doesn't stop me dreaming.

I mean I've got to, I mean if I don't then what's the point of me actually being here, what's the point of me writing and what's the point of me trying. If I don't have a dream I don't have a reason to fight and if I stop fighting then we all know how that's going to turn out, I don't ask for much out of life, I don't want tonnes of money because if I do I'll be dead within a year, I don't want flashy cars because they just don't interest me in the slightest, I don't want fake friends because I'm not in high-school anymore and quite frankly those days are behind me. I don't really want anything out of life except my friends, my family and just that little bit of peace and quiet. A place where I can just be free from the mess that goes on inside my mind. I mean that's not too much to ask for is it. I mean I want the simplest of simplest things, it's just that *he* interferes and when he interferes I'm screwed, I mean I am absolutely screwed, he's interfered twice in my life and the twice he's interfered it's nearly cost me my life, I don't like being at the bottom of the ocean, I don't like the cold, I don't like being able to see my friends but yet not get near them, I don't like reaching when I know I'm too far away to touch them. I hate the galoshes, I hate being trapped, I hate the feeling, the fear, the isolation and the pain. I hate the pain the most, I hate crying when I know that I'm trapped, I hate being trapped, I hate the fact that he is there laughing at me the whole time whilst I'm stuck there, I hate him laughing when I know it's him that's locked me there, I am his prisoner and until he says so I'm not moving, I am helpless, I am weak, fragile and at his mercy. I have no say, I have no power and worst of all I don't have the one thing that I need to face him, I don't have control. It's the control that's the worst, that and the cold, that and the fact that I know that I'm helpless to stop him, I know he can see me at the bottom, arms folded across my knees, staring helplessly, sobbing helplessly, sitting there at his beck and call, his mercy, it's his desire to keep me down that makes me want to get back up even more, I haven't named him, I refuse to name him, I'm happy leaving him as 'him', he'll always be 'he', it's bad enough when he comes to pay me a visit, it'd make me one hundred times worse if I named him, I don't want to name him, I don't want him in my life, why is he in my life, why does he want to put me there, why does he want to make me suffer? Why do I suffer? Why do I ache when this hits, why am I absolutely powerless to do anything about it? I pride myself on my ability to fight depression, it happens a lot more than people know. The fact that I fight it somedays without people knowing takes a lot of strength, it takes every single fibre of my being for me to do it but I do. I just get on with it and I do it. No-one asks for this, I certainly didn't, if it was up to me I'd stay as far away from this as possible, I hate it, it actually makes me want to vomit, I absolutely detest when it comes around, it's the cycle of it, the knowing that it's happening that's the worst. I touched on this earlier but that is by far the worst part of it, it makes me feel ill when I know it's coming. The blue sky is replaced with grey, the temperature drops and I feel the cold, I can manage but when I see that cliff and the water below then I know it's time to really brace myself, I know it's going to be ugly. How can I describe it accurately, can I describe it accurately? I don't know if I can. That's probably the best way I can surmise it. It's like someone reaches inside me and pulls every single emotion out of me apart from fear and even that gets numbed, the days where I feel nothing are by far the worst, they're a gut-wrench of a day, two days, three days, sometimes it lasts a week and then for no reason it disappears. It just ups and leaves me, it deserts me and leaves me wondering what happened, it leaves me asking why. I'm still asking why. It knocks me sideways. It's a total pain in the ass. (ass isn't swearing so it's not being counted as a swear...)

Psychologically though it does take it's toll, I don't feel the same for days, even though I feel lighter when it lifts I never feel myself again until about two days later, maybe even three days later. It's like a fatigue, it is fatigue because mentally I have to fight, I need to constantly fight so I'm absolutely and completely shattered. Fifteen years this has been going on, fifteen years so obviously there are going to be scars, that much is obvious but what I don't understand is why, I don't get why I have to go through this, why I have to endure psychological warfare, what ultimately is the fight, what's the cause of it? I certainly don't know but what I do know is this. That first day when I've got to be around people and I'm in a state of silence is the worst, I want to talk, I want to tell people not to worry about me but at the same time I can't, my mind is in silence and therefore I cannot speak unless I have to and by I have to I mean anything work related, anything else is a short, brief conversation. My mind allows it but no more. I spend two or three days almost in a state of razor-sharp focus, I am so efficient at work because it's all I can do. My productivity soars because it's all my mind will allow me to do. Believe me I have wanted to force myself out the other side but I dare not try, that's stepping into the unknown and quite frankly it's bad enough dealing with the mental silence, never mind the possibility of adding more things on top of it, I just don't see that ending well.

I'm sorry, I guess this is going a little bit deep, I am sorry if it's tough to read but believe me it's not much fun for me dealing with it, on my good days I am absolutely fantastic and on my bad days I'm just a wall of silence. The thing that annoys me the most by far are the good days that turn into bad days for no reason, the days where I'm coasting and then suddenly, 'BANG!' straight out of nowhere my mind capitulates, those are the days that I find hard to stomach, I don't deserve them, I don't think I deserve them, the bad days are bad enough, never mind having to have to unexpectedly deal with a bad day. They actually happen more than I'd like but thankfully they happen when I'm on my own so I can manage, when I'm out and they hit that's what I don't feel fair. When I'm out and I get hit *he* is the architect, I'm sure of it. He has to be otherwise why would it happen? I mean it's like a switch is flipped and that's it, I shut down and I have to leave, occasionally it's caused me to cry, this is walking through Glasgow by the way this isn't me on my own. I have to walk with my head up because in Glasgow I need to cross roads, on my own in the house is fine but I hate people seeing me cry. I'm pretty sure that's not normal, I think a lot of what I feel and experience is (relatively) normal but that isn't, that's not fair on me and certainly not on my friends who then worry. As I say I can take it, I'm a big boy I can take it on the chin but I don't think it's fair that my friends have to worry about me. That's not right and I don't like it one bit. Like all things though I just have to deal with it but then again that's what annoys me, even when I'm feeling close to my best I know I've always got to be on high-alert because I know somewhere in there it's lurking, prowling like a lion stalking a zebra, I know it's there because I feel it. Even on good days I'll be going about my business and just for a moment I know it's present, I can't see it, I can't pinpoint what's caused it but I damn sure know it's there. That right there is an annoyance, knowing that it's always somewhere in my mind, knowing it's watching and knowing it can strike me at any time, that's why I've got to always be extra vigilant. I don't want any surprises, I don't like when it comes out and surprises me, I can handle it on my own but when I'm with friends I can't, I have no time to prepare for it, I've got to just deal with it the best I can until I get home and then I can start to deal with it properly. I know what to do when I get home, I just don't like not having that level of control, I don't like being out of control and out of my mind at the same time, it makes me uncomfortable, it's too raw for me, it's like having my nerve endings exposed and the fear is touching them. It's painful, it's way too painful for me and it's too much to deal with me. It's when that strikes me I can sit and look out the window for hours, I can sit still for hours and focus on one flower, one tree, one car for hours at a time, I don't move, my hands stay clasped, my phone goes off and I don't respond, I don't even need to go to the toilet, I just sit, hands clasped looking, a blank stare across my face, my legs spread about two feet apart and all I do is stare, all I do is stare, I do nothing else, I just… sit. I'd love to say that after a few hours it goes away but it doesn't. That's the nice part of it, that's the good part of it. The bad part is when the thoughts start to swirl, the vortex opens and the hurricane starts heading towards me, I…am… powerless to stop it, I have no control over what it destroys, it just rips through my head like a hurricane through an old treehouse, nothing survives, it's best if I just lie there because if I try to fight it it just comes at me harder. I mean… it destroys everything, it takes everything I've built up and it just tears it apart like wet paper. I'm left with nothing again, I'm left there to go to sleep and just pick up the pieces, I mean I do, I start again, I have to start again because if I don't then my mood won't recover and I won't recover. I pick up the pieces because I believe that I'm strong, I have to believe in my strength and in my strength my belief is to build myself even stronger so when it comes again I'll have a better chance of my happiness staying intact. To my credit I am actually getting stronger and I do feel stronger but the big test is not when I'm feeling strong, it's when I'm at my weakest, THAT is the big test and then I have to see just how much I've built, I never outrun the vortex, there's no point trying because that happens, the big test is the hurricane that ensues, if I can come out of that with the foundations standing then I know I'm strong, I'm living in the belief that if I fight this battle long enough then eventually I'll be able to withstand the hurricane or maybe even the hurricane won't come my way. If the hurricane doesn't come my way then maybe I can avoid the vortex and if I avoid the vortex then maybe, just maybe I stand a chance of outrunning this and living my life as I see fit. That's the dream anyway, I don't know if that'll ever happen but I need to use the time I have to build again, I need to make use of this time so I can fortify, bolt and strengthen my mind because god knows when the next storm is coming, the last one I had was over a month ago so fingers crossed it's a long time before the next one hits. The dream is that another one doesn't hit but whether that happens or not we will just have to wait and see. Actually scrap that, I'll have to wait and see.

Should life be this hard? The short answer, nope. Then again I can't imagine my life being any other way, I know that's going to sound a bit….. bleugh but I genuinely can't see my life being lived in any other mindset, I think the logical answer way of looking at it is because I know no other way. I'm just fascinated by people though, I people watch a lot when I'm commuting, I do the same walking to work, I guess I'm just naturally curious, I always have been it's my way. I just like observing people, I should have worked in science instead of going down the call centre route, I could have been the shiz at behavioural studies, it could have been my wheelhouse, I could have made something of it. Watching and talking to people all day about their mind and what's in it, I think I might have just had a 'mindgasm', yea' I know that's pretty schoolyard humour wise but I am genuinely intrigued by people, not just their mind but their wee quriks, mannerisms and idiosyncrasies, I love them all, I love watching them, from people sorting their lunch to people turning a paper, I like seeing how people dress as well, it's all just one big people watch that I'm on. To an extent I do it when I'm out as well, watching people's behaviours change as the alcohol takes hold, it's inevitable but the change is quite fun to watch, well I'll rephrase that I'll do it until I get tipsy and then I just end up getting drunk and stagger home, it won't be the first time I've people watched whilst drunk and it won't be the last time. I guess what I'm trying to say is even though I feel I'm different to most people I'm still in love with people and how each and every person has almost perfectly unique mannerisms and behaviours. I'm sad that way, I think you're reading this going, 'ha, loser'. You might not be but it fascinates me, I'm up at 5am tomorrow for work and I'll guarantee you I do it on the train to work tomorrow. I don't think I actually stop people watching, it's actually quite fun when you see the same people every day depending on what shift I'm on. For example there's one guy who gets the train from Glasgow Queen Street to Charing Cross, he always reads a book and he always turns the page quite aggressively, I stand next to him on the train and he doesn't know I watch him... but I do. People are fun, try it. I try and pick up what different people do, especially with newspapers, some lick their thumb then turn the page, other people feather the page over. It's the same with typing, some people WHACK the keyboard, others tap tap tap, some touchtype and some you just can't hear. The more I write this the more I realise I'm really interested in people, I've always tried to keep my distance from people, especially women because I'm scared that if I get into a relationship then I'll get hurt. Now I know that sounds soppy as hell but it's true, I'm phenomenally scared to get involved because I'd have to something I never ever do, let people in. The sheer thought of that terrifies me, can I let someone in? I don't know if I can, I mean I want to but jeez, could I open up and talk? Can I open up and talk? I'd actually quite like to do that because I know I encourage people to talk things out. I'm there for people so maybe it could work. I'm scared though, it's a big step to take. I guess I'll have to take that one as it comes eh?

When I'm not people watching and I'm on the train I often sit and daydream out the window, I sit and I wonder what the future holds for me. I wonder what I'll be doing when I'm thirty four, the magical age of thirty five and beyond, what will I be like when I'm old? Where will I be career wise, where will I be staying? What will I actually look like in four years time, what will Glasgow look like, will I still be friends with the same people? I just sit and I ponder, I'll tell you one thing, it makes short work of the thirty minute commute from Larbert to Glasgow, it makes mincemeat of it. I get on the train and before I know it I'm in the tunnel at Queen Street although whenever I hit that tunnel I always fancy a nap, I have no idea why. It's the same when I have a few pints on my own, (not the nap part) I get lost in my own thoughts and I just tune out, before I know it fifteen minutes have past and I've finished my pint, I mean I completely and utterly tune out, it doesn't always happen but when it does it's quite nice, it's actually a really good place to be because it means I'm relaxed and when I'm relaxed I feel good, when I feel good...

.. well you get the idea where that's going.

Is any of this making sense? It makes sense to me because it's the inner workings of my head so I know what I'm saying, I don't know if it's translating across though, I hope it is because I want you to see what I see and feel what I feel through both good and bad. This for me is a journey, a journey that I didn't necessarily want to be on but one that regardless of how I feel I have to go through, sometimes there's beautiful sunshine, other times there are endless dark tunnels, I think it's too simplistic to say I've got to 'take the rough with the smooth', my journey's a lot more complicated than that and by the end of it I don't know what the outcome is going to be. I'd love to sit here and say that everything will be peachy but I know that's not true, I know ahead there are going to be really tough times and I know I'm going to need that build up of mental strength, god knows where I'm going to end up in terms of relationships. I mean I could end up getting married and having kids, well, not me having kids but you know what I mean with that. I mean that's something I've never even thought of, actually when I think about it there's a good reason that's never even entered my mind. I need to work on getting myself right first before I even consider entering a relationship and when I say 'getting myself right' I mean being in a position to be able to talk about anything that's not right i.e. bad days and the like. I mean for me it's hard to deal with never mind having someone else having to deal with it. I know if I meet the right person they'll love me regardless as I will with them but I'm not there just yet, maybe by the time I'm forty-three and all grey and the like. I don't know, I'm moving on though, that's definitely a worry/conversation for another day.

For any of my friends/family reading this I know it's hard, it's hard me writing this, after the first two I thought this would get easier but it doesn't. You guys need to know that I give this one hundred per cent and I am in a much better place than what I was back in December. For anyone outside friends and family reading this I don't know what your opinion is but I hope it gives you an insight into just how fragile and breakable the human mind can be. In my case it's a fine line between strength and breakage, it's a combination of a three inch thick steel vault door and a flimsy wooden door. It's not intentional it's just the way I am and it's something I need to manage. Before I close this off I need to address 'him'.

I don't know where he came from, I don't want to know where he came from but I'm trying so hard to control him. This is the first time I've actually been able to pinpoint exactly what I feel when the heaviness descends, I know somewhere I'm being watched and it scares me a little I'm not going to lie. Please believe me when I say I really don't like being so up and down, I mean I LOVE when I'm up and feeling great but doesn't everyone, it's just those days when he appears that I know I'm in trouble. Actually I've had enough of 'him', I don't want to think of it anymore tonight.

For anyone that suffers with depression I'd ask you to reach out, it's by far the hardest thing you will ever have to do but it's totally worth it. You don't need to suffer in silence, it is by far the greatest mistake you can make, I'm talking from experience because for months I hid it and it nearly cost me my life, talk to someone, anyone about it. Call 'The Samaritans', phone someone, speak to a friend, the sooner you can talk about it the better you will feel. Although for me it was hard and I ended up crying I did eventually manage to talk to someone and I did feel better, I ended up with a great support network but I nearly left it too late, I waited way too late before asking for help. Please please please don't ever be afraid to ask for help, speak to your GP, they're there for you and will support you one hundred percent, go online and search mental health forums, talking online can be just as effective, I would encourage anyone reading this who has any mental health issue to seek advice when they can. It's not as easy as that, I know but there are people that care, your friends care and there are kind people out there who are by your side. You're not alone, never think that you are. That being said I know how it feels, I've used words like 'trapped' and 'abyss' and that's exactly what it feels like, it feels like an absolute hole you're down and there's no escaping, it is the absolute worst place to be and unless you speak to someone that understands they won't be able to help you. I count myself really lucky because my best friend went through the exact same thing at the exact same time and I couldn't have made it this far without her. She helped me so much when I was at my worst, she was there when I was walking about all the time with a pair of yellow sunglasses on all the time, they were my way of hiding, she's been there for me through thick and thin and I love her to bits, I've always counted myself really lucky because I somehow end up with amazing people in my life, I'm not really sure I deserve them but I'm glad I have them, I'm definitely a people person and I've been there for more than my fair share, I've laughed with friends, cried with friends, hung out with friends and got drunk with friends, if I had a choice between having a million pounds or my friends what would I choose?

God the money, you wouldn't see me for dust! I kid, I'd choose my friends because they're loyal to me and I'm loyal to them, I am nothing without the right people in my life. I've denied this for years but I *need* people in my life, I need the banter, the conversations and the company, although I need time to myself I'll crumble if I don't have my friends, they are the ones who give me strength, they're the ones I know I can count on if I'm having a bad day, they're the ones that pick me up and carry me until I feel better and vice versa. Friends are a wonderful thing, people are a wonderful thing, never ever underestimate the awesomeness of people, you'd be surprised at just how awesome the right people are, they are fantastic human beings. I also have a fantastic family, I don't know where I'd be without their support, they have done so much for me and I am eternally grateful for all that they do for me, I've now learned that if I'm having a not so good time then I can talk to them, I know that they are behind me and talking to them isn't a sign of weakness, it's a sign of strength that I recognise that I can talk to them, I've said it before and I'll say it again, don't be afraid to talk to people that share the same fears as you, you might surprise yourself by what you find.

Underneath all of this I am actually quite a simple guy, all I really want to do is the usual kind of stuff that a guy my age does, after work go and meet my friends, dance the night away in Rufus T Firefly/Solid Rock and listen to some good old fashioned rock and roll, I love music, I love going to gigs, I love my friends, I LOVE my friends, I ABSOLUTELY FRICKIN' ADORE MY FRIENDS, I am surrounded by great people, I'm surrounded by a great family and although they don't know half of what I actually go through they should know this. They mean the absolute world to me and I want them to know until the day I die I will love them ten thousand times more than they will ever love me. I want them to know that they are my world and without them my world is dark, without them I am forever locked in a basement with a blindfold on and no way of getting out, without them I do not have the strength to go on, I do not have a direction, without them I am well and truly fooked. Without everyone around me the world is a much darker and scarier place, without them I am nothing, with them I am everything, I fly, I soar and I believe, I breathe, I believe, I breathe and I believe. I am all that I can be with them behind me, they are my world, my rock and my strength. Without you I am merely a human, with you I can be me, with you my struggles have a light, without you I'm lost, floundering in the abyss, it's five hundred miles wide and I'm looking for a key, it's pitch black without you guys, with you beside me I am so much greater than what I am on my own. I feed off of your strength and your love, you're loving me propels me, it pushes me to be better, it pushes me to work harder, with you I am invincible, bulletproof and the definition of resiliency, without you I am unprotected and alone. I cannot live without you guys and if I don't have you guys... I cannot live, I am a flower starved of light and water, I will wither and die. I will disappear, wander and die. I will be mourned and forgotten, I will be a memory without you, I will always be with you but in spirit and mind, not in person. I need you, I am nothing without you, you guys are what drive me to beat this and I need you, I cannot do this without you, stay behind me, I need your strength for when mines fades. I love you, I don't say it enough but I love you more than I could ever speak or write, I love you unconditionally, I love you with faults, with anomalies, inconsistencies and flaws, I love you all and I always will. I just... find it hard to say that, it's what I feel, it's all I feel, I have so much love for everyone in my life but I can never say it. I want to say it but I just can't, it's not the done thing to just blurt out to someone that you love them.

I don't want to disappear, I don't want to wither and die, I want to fight this again and I want to beat this, I want to enjoy myself and I want to be surrounded by the people I love the most, I know I'm not on my own with this, I know that but it's hard trying to open up with something you've been fighting on your own. The amount of times I have lay in bed crying over my inability to talk you wouldn't believe, the amount of times I have stared at myself in the mirror and tried to find something to believe in. I fight so hard and I fight all the time, I constantly fight this but it gets tiring, it gets so unbelievably tiring. That's why I need those around me, I need them for what lies ahead of me, for what I'm going to face. If I have my friends and family by my side then I have a chance, I NEED you a hell of a lot more than you will ever need me. You guys actually have no idea what you mean to me, I could write one hundred thousand words and I probably couldn't even scratch the surface of what you mean to me. I love you with all my heart and even though I'm inevitably going to have bad days, that doesn't mean that every day is going to be a bad day. Guys you need to understand that this cripples me, I mean emotionally and mentally it absolutely cripples me. I've been to hell, it's nothing special. Let's make a lifetime of memories and when we're all old and grey we can look back and laugh at all we went through. Let's make this the start of something beautiful.

Thank you so much for reading.

Dave Roberts